The New Air Fryer Recipe Book

Cook with Simple, Tasty and Wholesome Ingredients

By

Caroline Taylor

All rights reserved. Copyright 2020.

Table of content

Authentic Mediterranean Calamari Salad..1

Buttermilk Tuna fillets 3

Cajun Cod Fillets with Avocado Sauce 6

Cajun Fish Cakes with Cheese 9

Coconut Shrimp with Orange Sauce 12

Cod and Shallot Frittata...15

Crab Cake Burgers 17

Crispy Mustardy Fish Fingers 20

Crispy Tilapia Fillets...23

Delicious Snapper en Papillote...26

Dilled and Glazed Salmon Steaks 29

Easy Lobster Tails 32

Easy Prawns alla Parmigiana..35

English-Style Flounder Fillets 38

Greek-Style Roast Fish..41

Grilled Hake with Garlic Sauce 44

Grilled Salmon Steaks 47

Grilled Tilapia with Portobello Mushrooms...50

Halibut Cakes with Horseradish Mayo...53

Indian Famous Fish Curry 56

Korean-Style Salmon Patties 59

Monkfish Fillets with Romano Cheese 62

Monkfish with Sautéed Vegetables and Olives 64

Old Bay Calamari 67

Quick-Fix Seafood Breakfast 70

Salmon Filets with Fennel Slaw 73

Salmon with Baby Bok Choy 75

Saucy Garam Masala Fish 78

Scallops with Pineapple Salsa and Pickled Onions 80

Seed-Crusted Codfish Fillets 82

Shrimp Scampi Linguine 84

Smoked Halibut and Eggs in Brioche 86

Snapper Casserole with Gruyere Cheese 88

Spicy Curried King Prawns 90

Sunday Fish with Sticky Sauce 92

Swordfish with Roasted Peppers and Garlic Sauce 94

Tortilla-Crusted Haddock Fillets 96

Tuna Steak with Roasted Cherry Tomatoes 98

Tuna Steaks with Pearl Onions 100

Vermouth and Garlic Shrimp Skewers 102

Alphabetical Index 104

Authentic Mediterranean Calamari Salad

(Ready in about 15 minutes | Servings 3)

Per serving:

457 Calories; 31.3g Fat; 18.4g Carbs; 25.1g Protein; 9.2g Sugars

Ingredients

1 pound squid, cleaned, sliced into rings 2 tablespoons sherry wine

1/2 teaspoon granulated garlic Salt, to taste

1/2 teaspoon ground black pepper 1/2 teaspoon basil

1/2 teaspoon dried rosemary

1 cup grape tomatoes

1 small red onion, thinly sliced

1/3 cup Kalamata olives, pitted and sliced 1/2 cup mayonnaise

1 teaspoon yellow mustard

1/2 cup fresh flat-leaf parsley leaves, coarsely chopped

Directions

Start by preheating the Air Fryer to 400 degrees F. Spritz the Air Fryer basket with cooking oil.

Toss the squid rings with the sherry wine, garlic, salt, pepper, basil, and rosemary. Cook in the preheated Air Fryer for 5 minutes, shaking the basket halfway through the cooking time.

Work in batches and let it cool to room temperature. When the squid is cool enough, add the remaining Ingredients.

Gently stir to combine and serve well chilled. Bon appétit!

Buttermilk Tuna fillets

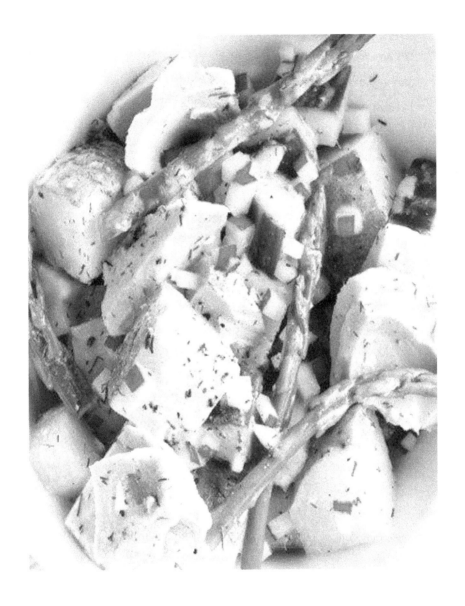

(Ready in about 50 minutes | Servings 3)

Per serving:

266 Calories; 5.7g Fat; 13.6g Carbs; 37.8g Protein; 2.5g Sugars

Ingredients

1 pound tuna fillets 1/2 cup buttermilk

1/2 cup tortilla chips, crushed

1/4 cup parmesan cheese, grated 1/4 cup cassava flour

Salt and ground black pepper, to taste

1 teaspoon mustard seeds 1 teaspoon paprika

1 teaspoon garlic powder

1/2 teaspoon onion powder

Directions

Place the tuna fillets and buttermilk in a bowl; cover and let it sit for 30 minutes.

In a shallow bowl, thoroughly combine the remaining Ingredients; mix until well combined.

Dip the tuna fillets in the parmesan mixture until they are covered on all sides.

Cook in the preheated Air Fryer at 380 degrees F for 12 minutes, turning halfway through the cooking time. Bon appétit!

Cajun Cod Fillets with Avocado Sauce

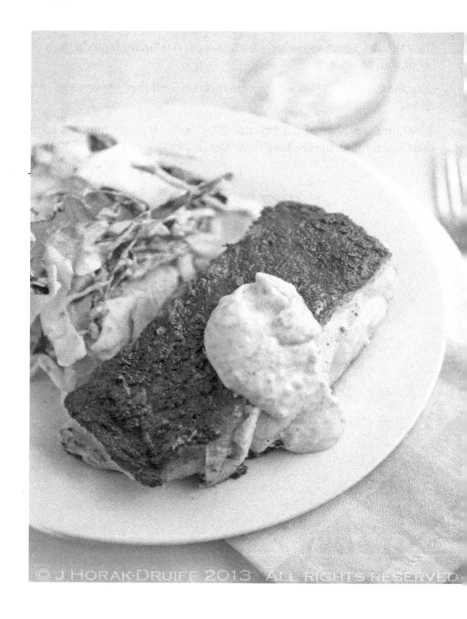

(Ready in about 20 minutes | Servings 2)

Per serving:

418 Calories; 22.7g Fat; 12.5g Carbs; 40.1g Protein; 0.9g Sugars

Ingredients

2 cod fish fillets 1 egg

Sea salt, to taste

1/2 cup tortilla chips, crushed 2 teaspoons olive oil

1/2 avocado, peeled, pitted, and mashed

1 tablespoon mayonnaise 3 tablespoons sour cream

1/2 teaspoon yellow mustard

1 teaspoon lemon juice 1 garlic clove, minced

1/4 teaspoon black pepper

1/4 teaspoon salt

1/4 teaspoon hot pepper sauce

Directions

Start by preheating your Air Fryer to 360 degrees F. Spritz the Air Fryer basket with cooking oil.

Pat dry the fish fillets with a kitchen towel. Beat the egg in a shallow bowl.

In a separate bowl, thoroughly combine the salt, crushed tortilla chips, and olive oil.

Dip the fish into the egg, then, into the crumb mixture, making sure to coat thoroughly. Cook in the preheated Air Fryer approximately 12 minutes.

Meanwhile, make the avocado sauce by mixing the remaining Ingredients in a bowl. Place in your refrigerator until ready to serve.

Serve the fish fillets with chilled avocado sauce on the side. Bon appétit!

Cajun Fish Cakes with Cheese

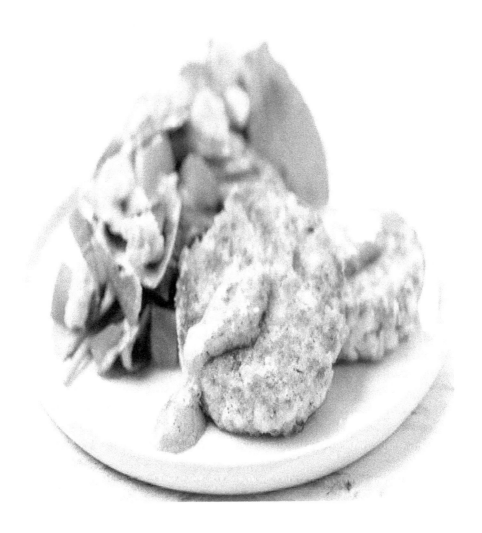

(Ready in about 30 minutes | Servings 4)

Per serving:

478 Calories; 30.1g Fat; 27.2g Carbs; 23.8g Protein; 2g Sugars

Ingredients

2 catfish fillets

1 cup all-purpose flour 3 ounces butter

1 teaspoon baking powder 1 teaspoon baking soda 1/2 cup buttermilk

1 teaspoon Cajun seasoning 1 cup Swiss cheese, shredded

Directions

Bring a pot of salted water to a boil. Boil the fish fillets for 5 minutes or until it is opaque. Flake the fish into small pieces.

Mix the remaining Ingredients in a bowl; add the fish and mix until well combined. Shape the fish mixture into 12 patties.

Cook in the preheated Air Fryer at 380 degrees F for 15 minutes. Work in batches. Enjoy!

Coconut Shrimp with Orange Sauce

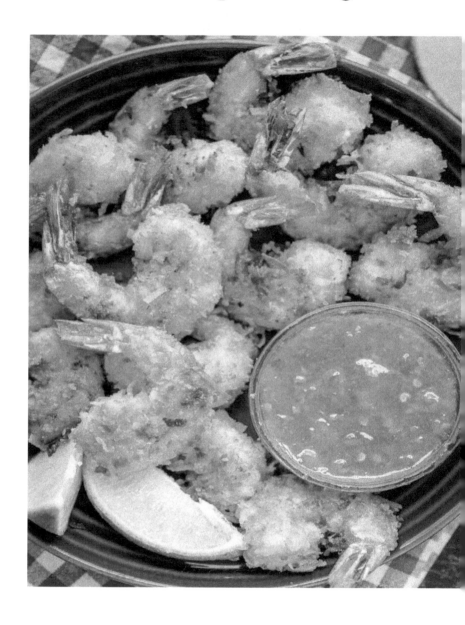

(Ready in about 1 hour 30 minutes | Servings 3)

Per serving:

487 Calories; 21.7g Fat; 35.9g Carbs; 37.6g Protein; 8.4g Sugars

Ingredients

1 pound shrimp, cleaned and deveined Sea salt and white pepper, to taste

1/2 cup all-purpose flour

1 egg

1/4 cup shredded coconut, unsweetened 3/2 cup fresh bread crumbs

2 tablespoons olive oil

1 lemon, cut into wedges

Dipping Sauce:

2 tablespoons butter 1/2 cup orange juice

2 tablespoons soy sauce A pinch of salt

1/2 teaspoon tapioca starch

2 tablespoons fresh parsley, minced

Directions

Pat dry the shrimp and season them with salt and white pepper.

Place the flour on a large tray; then, whisk the egg in a shallow bowl. In a third shallow bowl, place the shredded coconut and breadcrumbs.

Dip the shrimp in the flour, then, dip in the egg. Lastly, coat the shrimp with the shredded coconut and bread crumbs. Refrigerate for 1 hour.

Then, transfer to the cooking basket. Drizzle with olive oil and cook in the preheated Air Fryer at 370 degrees F for 6 minutes. Work in batches.

Meanwhile, melt the butter in a small saucepan over medium-high heat; add the orange juice and bring it to a boil; reduce the heat and allow it to simmer approximately 7 minutes.

Add the soy sauce, salt, and tapioca; continue simmering until the sauce has thickened and reduced. Spoon the sauce over the shrimp and garnish with lemon wedges and parsley. Serve immediately.

Cod and Shallot Frittata

(Ready in about 20 minutes | Servings 3)

Per serving:

454 Calories; 30.8g Fat; 10.3g Carbs; 32.4g Protein; 4.1g Sugars

Ingredients

2 cod fillets

6 eggs

1/2 cup milk

1 shallot, chopped

2 garlic cloves, minced

Sea salt and ground black pepper, to taste 1/2 teaspoon red pepper flakes, crushed

Directions

Bring a pot of salted water to a boil. Boil the cod fillets for 5 minutes or until it is opaque. Flake the fish into bite-sized pieces.

In a mixing bowl, whisk the eggs and milk. Stir in the shallots, garlic, salt, black pepper, and red pepper flakes. Stir in the reserved fish.

Pour the mixture into the lightly greased baking pan.

Cook in the preheated Air Fryer at 360 degrees F for 9 minutes, flipping over halfway through. Bon appétit!

Crab Cake Burgers

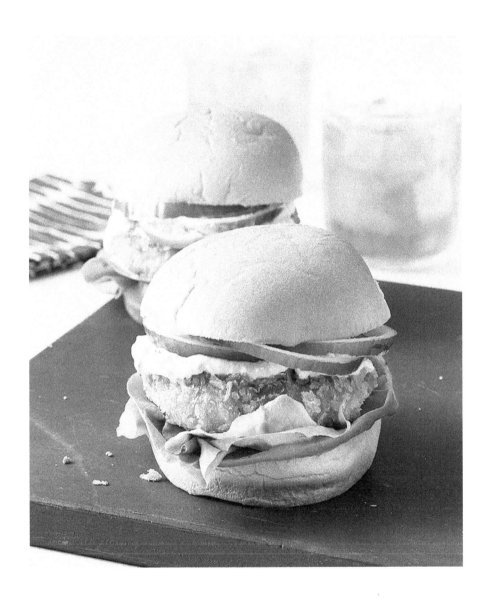

(Ready in about 2 hours 20 minutes | Servings 3)

Per serving:

500 Calories; 15.1g Fat; 51g Carbs; 44.3g Protein; 1.7g Sugars

Ingredients

2 eggs, beaten

1 shallot, chopped

2 garlic cloves, crushed 1 tablespoon olive oil

1 teaspoon yellow mustard

1 teaspoon fresh cilantro, chopped 10 ounces crab meat

1 cup tortilla chips, crushed 1/2 teaspoon cayenne pepper

1/2 teaspoon ground black pepper Sea salt, to taste

3/4 cup fresh bread crumbs

Directions

In a mixing bowl, thoroughly combine the eggs, shallot, garlic, olive oil, mustard, cilantro, crab meat, tortilla chips, cayenne pepper, black pepper, and salt. Mix until well combined.

Shape the mixture into 6 patties. Dip the crab patties into the fresh breadcrumbs, coating well on all sides. Place in your refrigerator for 2 hours.

Spritz the crab patties with cooking oil on both sides. Cook in the preheated Air Fryer at 360 degrees F for 14 minutes. Serve on dinner rolls if desired. Bon appétit!

Crispy Mustardy Fish Fingers

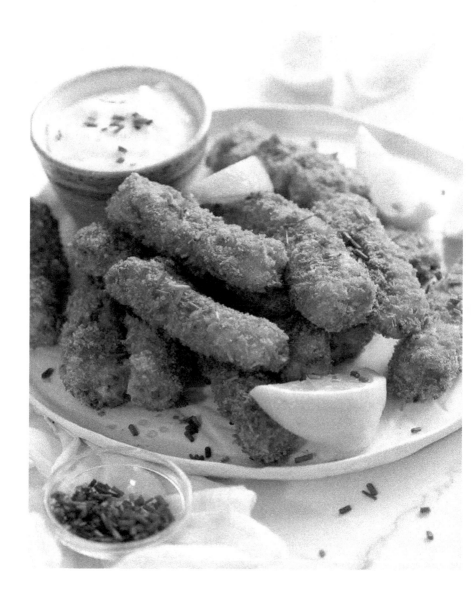

(Ready in about 20 minutes | Servings 4)

Per serving:

468 Calories; 12.7g Fat; 45.6g Carbs; 41.9g Protein; 1.4g Sugars

Ingredients

1 ½ pounds tilapia pieces (fingers) 1/2 cup all-purpose flour

2 eggs

1 tablespoon yellow mustard 1 cup cornmeal

1 teaspoon garlic powder

1 teaspoon onion powder

Sea salt and ground black pepper, to taste 1/2 teaspoon celery powder

2 tablespoons peanut oil

Directions

Pat dry the fish fingers with a kitchen towel.

To make a breading station, place the all-purpose flour in a shallow dish. In a separate dish, whisk the eggs with mustard.

In a third bowl, mix the remaining Ingredients.

Dredge the fish fingers in the flour, shaking the excess into the bowl; dip in the egg mixture and turn to coat evenly; then, dredge in the cornmeal mixture, turning a couple of times to coat evenly.

Cook in the preheated Air Fryer at 390 degrees F for 5 minutes; turn them over and cook another 5 minutes. Enjoy!

Crispy Tilapia Fillets

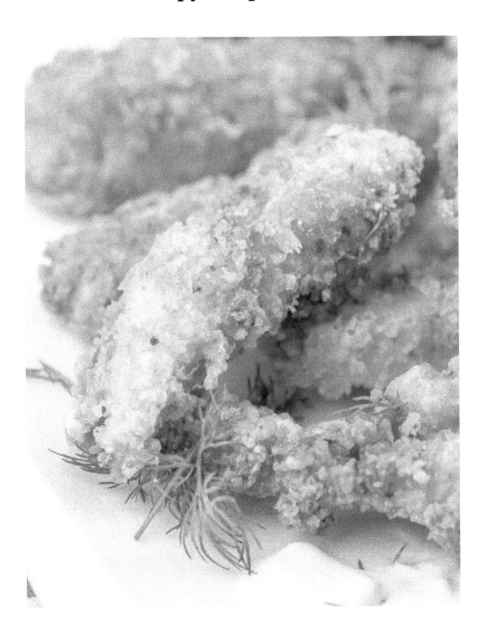

(Ready in about 20 minutes | Servings 5)

Per serving:

315 Calories; 9.1g Fat; 19.4g Carbs; 38.5g Protein; 0.7g Sugars

Ingredients

5 tablespoons all-purpose flour Sea salt and white pepper, to taste 1 teaspoon garlic paste

2 tablespoons extra virgin olive oil 1/2 cup cornmeal

5 tilapia fillets, slice into halves

Directions

Combine the flour, salt, white pepper, garlic paste, olive oil, and cornmeal in a Ziploc bag. Add the fish fillets and shake to coat well.

Spritz the Air Fryer basket with cooking spray. Cook in the preheated Air Fryer at 400 degrees F for 10 minutes; turn them over and cook for 6 minutes more. Work in batches.

Serve with lemon wedges if desired. Enjoy!

Delicious Snapper en Papillote

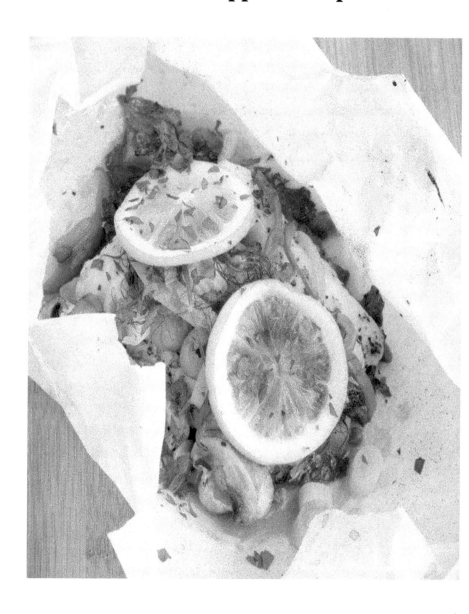

(Ready in about 20 minutes | Servings 2)

Per serving:

329 Calories; 9.8g Fat; 12.7g Carbs; 46.7g Protein; 5.4g Sugars

Ingredients

2 snapper fillets

1 shallot, peeled and sliced 2 garlic cloves, halved

1 bell pepper, sliced

1 small-sized serrano pepper, sliced 1 tomato, sliced

1 tablespoon olive oil

1/4 teaspoon freshly ground black pepper 1/2 teaspoon paprika

Sea salt, to taste 2 bay leaves

Directions

Place two parchment sheets on a working surface. Place the fish in the center of one side of the parchment paper.

Top with the shallot, garlic, peppers, and tomato. Drizzle olive oil over the fish and vegetables. Season with black pepper, paprika, and salt. Add the bay leaves.

Fold over the other half of the parchment. Now, fold the paper around the edges tightly and create a half moon shape, sealing the fish inside.

Cook in the preheated Air Fryer at 390 degrees F for 15 minutes. Serve warm.

Dilled and Glazed Salmon Steaks

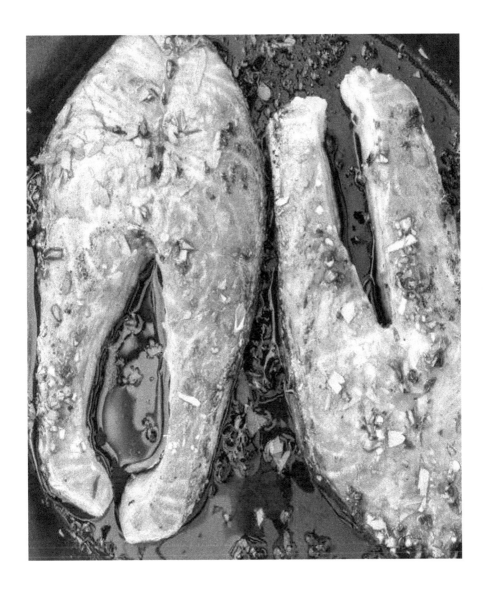

(Ready in about 20 minutes | Servings 2)

Per serving:

421 Calories; 16.8g Fat; 19.9g Carbs; 46.7g Protein; 18.1g Sugars

Ingredients

2 salmon steaks Coarse sea salt, to taste

1/4 teaspoon freshly ground black pepper, or more to taste

2 tablespoons honey

1 tablespoon sesame oil Zest of 1 lemon

1 tablespoon fresh lemon juice 1 teaspoon garlic, minced

1/2 teaspoon smoked cayenne pepper

1/2 teaspoon dried dill

Directions

Preheat your Air Fryer to 380 degrees F. Pat dry the salmon steaks with a kitchen towel.

In a ceramic dish, combine the remaining Ingredients until everything is well whisked.

Add the salmon steaks to the ceramic dish and let them sit in the refrigerator for 1 hour. Now, place the salmon steaks in the cooking basket. Reserve the marinade.

Cook for 12 minutes, flipping halfway through the cooking time.

Meanwhile, cook the marinade in a small sauté pan over a moderate flame. Cook until the sauce has thickened.

Pour the sauce over the steaks and serve with mashed potatoes if desired. Bon appétit!

Easy Lobster Tails

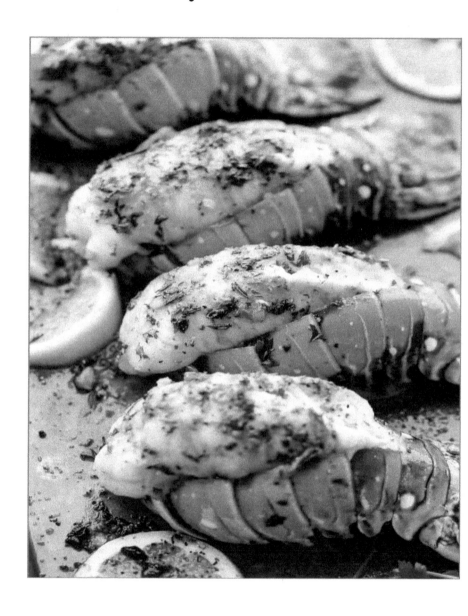

(Ready in about 20 minutes | Servings 5)

Per serving:

422 Calories; 7.9g Fat; 49.9g Carbs; 35.4g Protein; 3.1g Sugars

Ingredients

2 pounds fresh lobster tails, cleaned and halved, in shells 2 tablespoons butter, melted

1 teaspoon onion powder

1 teaspoon cayenne pepper

Salt and ground black pepper, to taste 2 garlic cloves, minced

1 cup cornmeal

1 cup green olives

Directions

In a plastic closeable bag, thoroughly combine all Ingredients; shake to combine well.

Transfer the coated lobster tails to the greased cooking basket.

Cook in the preheated Air Fryer at 390 degrees for 6 to 7 minutes, shaking the basket halfway through. Work in batches.

Serve with green olives and enjoy!

Easy Prawns alla Parmigiana

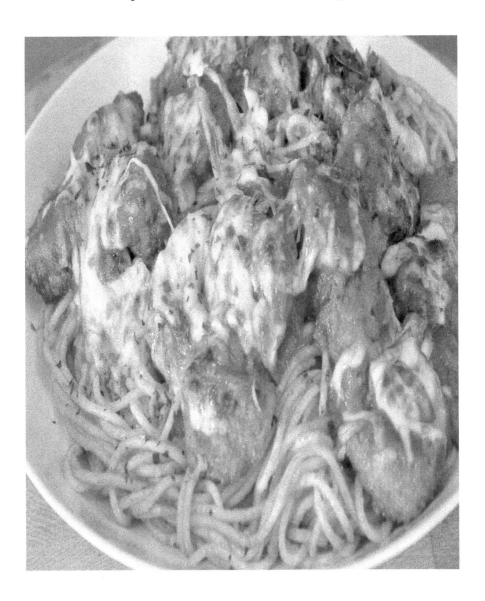

(Ready in about 20 minutes | Servings 4)

Per serving:

442 Calories; 10.3g Fat; 40.4g Carbs; 43.7g Protein; 1.2g Sugars

Ingredients

2 egg whites

1 cup all-purpose flour

1 cup Parmigiano-Reggiano, grated 1/2 cup fine breadcrumbs

1/2 teaspoon celery seeds 1/2 teaspoon porcini powder 1/2 teaspoon onion powder 1 teaspoon garlic powder 1/2 teaspoon dried rosemary 1/2 teaspoon sea salt

1/2 teaspoon ground black pepper 1 ½ pounds prawns, deveined

Directions

To make a breading station, whisk the egg whites in a shallow dish. In a separate dish, place the all-purpose flour.

In a third dish, thoroughly combine the Parmigiano-Reggiano, breadcrumbs, and seasonings; mix to combine well.

Dip the prawns in the flour, then, into the egg whites; lastly, dip them in the parm/breadcrumb mixture. Roll until they are covered on all sides.

Cook in the preheated Air Fryer at 390 degrees F for 5 to 7 minutes or until golden brown. Work in batches. Serve with lemon wedges if desired.

English-Style Flounder Fillets

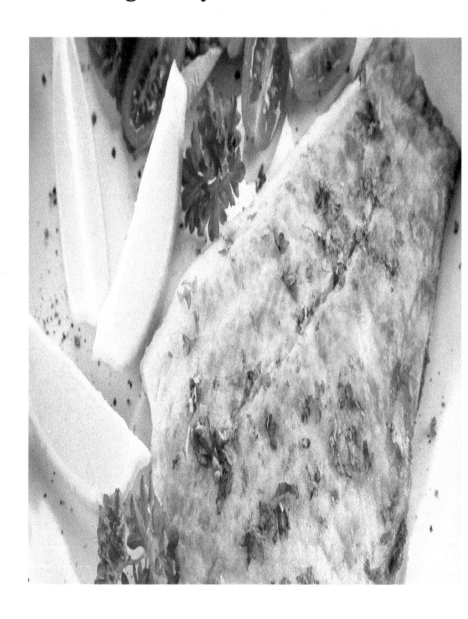

(Ready in about 20 minutes | Servings 2)

Per serving:

432 Calories; 16.7g Fat; 29g Carbs; 38.4g Protein; 2.7g Sugars

Ingredients

2 flounder fillets

1/4 cup all-purpose flour 1 egg

1/2 teaspoon Worcestershire sauce 1/2 cup bread crumbs

1/2 teaspoon lemon pepper

1/2 teaspoon coarse sea salt 1/4 teaspoon chili powder

Directions

Rinse and pat dry the flounder fillets. Place the flour in a large pan.

Whisk the egg and Worcestershire sauce in a shallow bowl. In a separate bowl, mix the bread crumbs with the lemon pepper, salt, and chili powder.

Dredge the fillets in the flour, shaking off the excess. Then, dip them into the egg mixture. Lastly, coat the fish fillets with the breadcrumb mixture until they are coated on all sides.

Spritz with cooking spray and transfer to the Air Fryer basket. Cook at 390 degrees for 7 minutes.

Turn them over, spritz with cooking spray on the other side, and cook another 5 minutes. Bon appétit!

Greek-Style Roast Fish

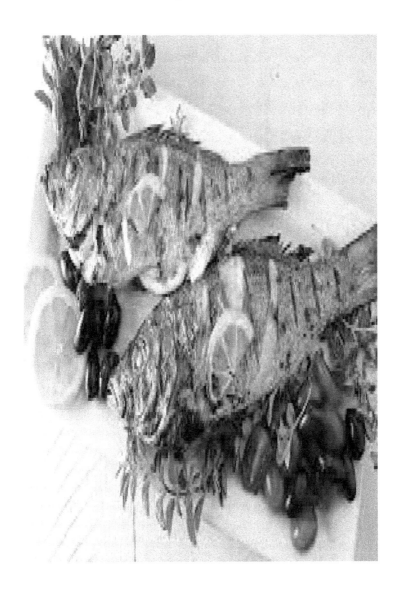

(Ready in about 20 minutes | Servings 3)

Per serving:

345 Calories; 32.7g Fat; 8.4g Carbs; 45.9g Protein; 3.5g Sugars

Ingredients

2 tablespoons olive oil 1 red onion, sliced

2 cloves garlic, chopped

1 Florina pepper, deveined and minced 3 pollock fillets, skinless

2 ripe tomatoes, diced

12 Kalamata olives, pitted and chopped 2 tablespoons capers

1 teaspoon oregano

1 teaspoon rosemary Sea salt, to taste

1/2 cup white wine

Directions

Start by preheating your Air Fryer to 360 degrees F. Heat the oil in a baking pan. Once hot, sauté the onion, garlic, and pepper for 2 to 3 minutes or until fragrant.

Add the fish fillets to the baking pan. Top with the tomatoes, olives, and capers. Sprinkle with the oregano, rosemary, and salt. Pour in white wine and transfer to the cooking basket.

Turn the temperature to 395 degrees F and bake for 10 minutes. Taste for seasoning and serve on individual plates, garnished with some extra Mediterranean herbs if desired. Enjoy!

Grilled Hake with Garlic Sauce

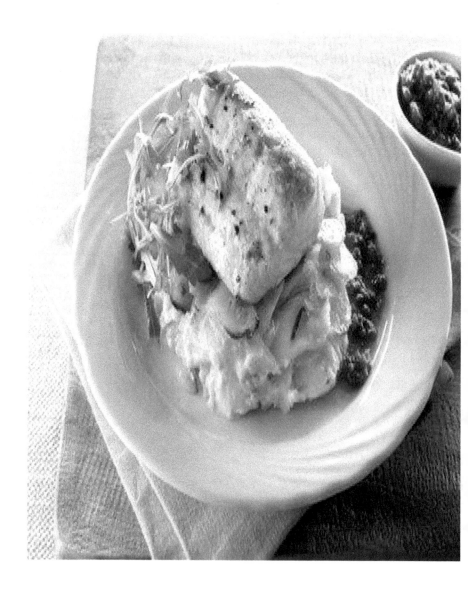

(Ready in about 20 minutes | Servings 3)

Per serving:

479 Calories; 22g Fat; 29.1g Carbs; 39.1g Protein; 3.6g Sugars

Ingredients

3 hake fillets

6 tablespoons mayonnaise 1 teaspoon Dijon mustard

1 tablespoon fresh lime juice 1 cup panko crumbs

Salt, to taste

1/4 teaspoon ground black pepper, or more to taste Garlic Sauce

1/4 cup Greek-style yogurt

2 tablespoons olive oil 2 cloves garlic, minced

1/2 teaspoon tarragon leaves, minced

Directions

Pat dry the hake fillets with a kitchen towel.

In a shallow bowl, whisk together the mayo, mustard, and lime juice. In another shallow bowl, thoroughly combine the panko crumbs with salt, and black pepper.

Spritz the Air Fryer grill pan with non-stick cooking spray. Grill in the preheated Air Fry at 395 degrees F for 10 minutes, flipping halfway through the cooking time.

Serve immediately.

Grilled Salmon Steaks

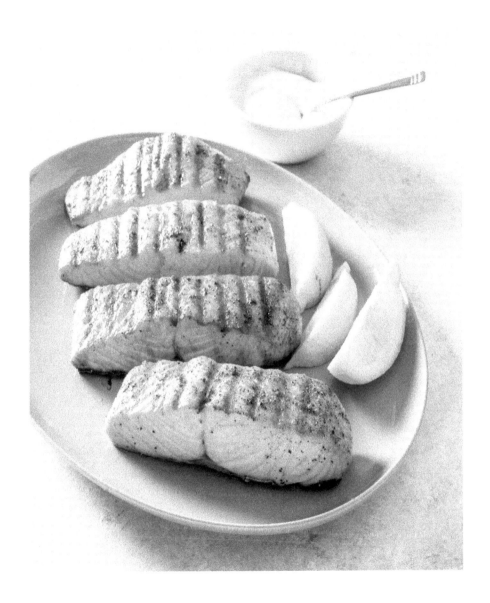

(Ready in about 45 minutes | Servings 4)

Per serving:

420 Calories; 23g Fat; 2.5g Carbs; 48.5g Protein; 0.7g Sugars

Ingredients

2 cloves garlic, minced

4 tablespoons butter, melted

Sea salt and ground black pepper, to taste 1 teaspoon smoked paprika

1/2 teaspoon onion powder 1 tablespoon lime juice

1/4 cup dry white wine 4 salmon steaks

Directions

Place all Ingredients in a large ceramic dish. Cover and let it marinate for 30 minutes in the refrigerator.

Arrange the salmon steaks on the grill pan. Bake at 390 degrees for 5 minutes, or until the salmon steaks are easily flaked with a fork.

Flip the fish steaks, baste with the reserved marinade, and cook another 5 minutes. Bon appétit!

Grilled Tilapia with Portobello Mushrooms

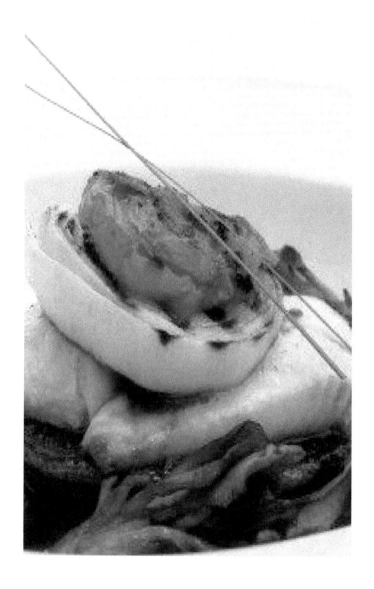

(Ready in about 20 minutes | Servings 2)

Per serving:

320 Calories; 11.4g Fat; 29.1g Carbs; 49.3g Protein; 4.2g Sugars

Ingredients

2 tilapia fillets

1 tablespoon avocado oil

1/2 teaspoon red pepper flakes, crushed 1/2 teaspoon dried sage, crushed

1/4 teaspoon lemon pepper 1/2 teaspoon sea salt

1 teaspoon dried parsley flakes

4 medium-sized Portobello mushrooms A few drizzles of liquid smoke

Directions

Toss all Ingredients in a mixing bowl; except for the mushrooms.

Transfer the tilapia fillets to a lightly greased grill pan. Preheat your Air Fryer to 400 degrees F and cook the tilapia fillets for 5 minutes.

Now, turn the fillets over and add the Portobello mushrooms. Continue to cook for 5 minutes longer or until mushrooms are tender and the fish is opaque. Serve immediately.

Halibut Cakes with Horseradish Mayo

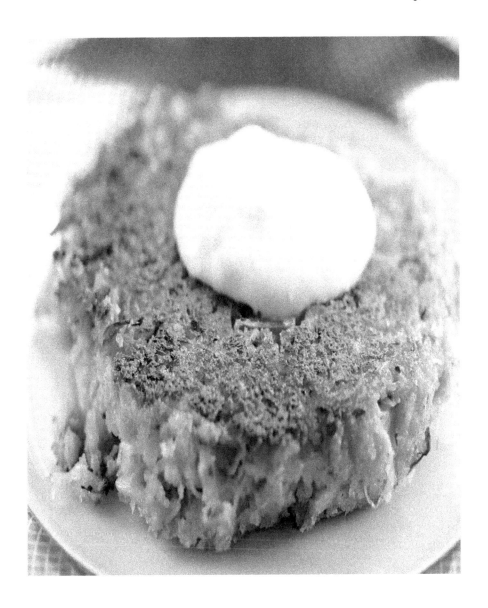

(Ready in about 20 minutes | Servings 4)

Per serving:

470 Calories; 38.2g Fat; 6.3g Carbs; 24.4g Protein; 1.5g Sugars

Ingredients

Halibut Cakes:

1 pound halibut

2 tablespoons olive oil

1/2 teaspoon cayenne pepper 1/4 teaspoon black pepper Salt, to taste

2 tablespoons cilantro, chopped 1 shallot, chopped

2 garlic cloves, minced

1/2 cup Romano cheese, grated 1/2 cup breadcrumbs

1 egg, whisked

1 tablespoon Worcestershire sauce Mayo Sauce:

1 teaspoon horseradish, grated

1/2 cup mayonnaise

Directions

Start by preheating your Air Fryer to 380 degrees F. Spritz the Air Fryer basket with cooking oil.

Mix all Ingredients for the halibut cakes in a bowl; knead with your hands until everything is well incorporated.

Shape the mixture into equally sized patties. Transfer your patties to the Air Fryer basket. Cook the fish patties for 10 minutes, turning them over halfway through.

Mix the horseradish and mayonnaise. Serve the halibut cakes with the horseradish mayo. Bon appétit!

Indian Famous Fish Curry

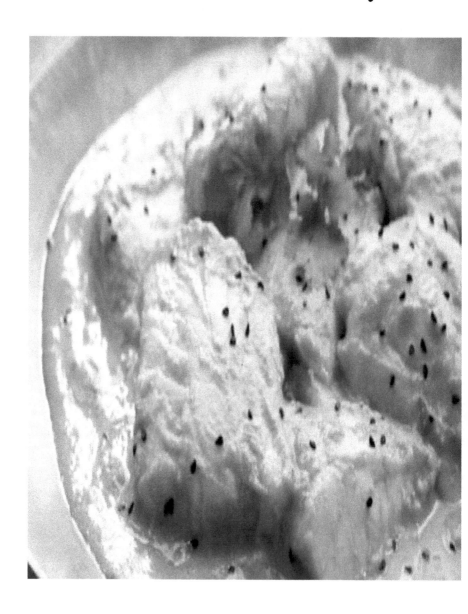

(Ready in about 25 minutes | Servings 4)

Per serving:

449 Calories; 29.1g Fat; 20.4g Carbs; 27.3g Protein; 13.3g Sugars

Ingredients

2 tablespoons sunflower oil 1/2 pound fish, chopped

2 red chilies, chopped

1 tablespoon coriander powder 1 teaspoon curry paste

1 cup coconut milk

Salt and white pepper, to taste 1/2 teaspoon fenugreek seeds 1 shallot, minced

1 garlic clove, minced 1 ripe tomato, pureed

Directions

Preheat your Air Fryer to 380 degrees F; brush the cooking basket with 1 tablespoon of sunflower oil.

Cook your fish for 10 minutes on both sides. Transfer to the baking pan that is previously greased with the remaining tablespoon of sunflower oil.

Add the remaining Ingredients and reduce the heat to 350 degrees F. Continue to cook an additional 10 to 12 minutes or until everything is heated through. Enjoy!

Korean-Style Salmon Patties

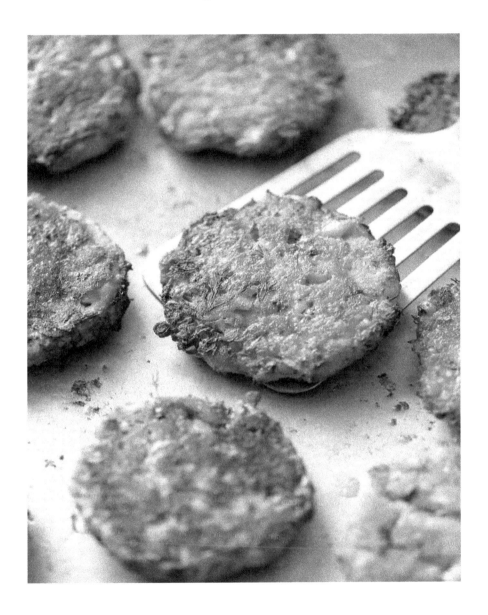

(Ready in about 15 minutes | Servings 4)

Per serving:

396 Calories; 20.1g Fat; 16.7g Carbs; 35.2g Protein; 3.1g Sugars

Ingredients

1 pound salmon

1 egg

1 garlic clove, minced 2 green onions, minced 1/2 cup rolled oats Sauce:

1 teaspoon rice wine

1 ½ tablespoons soy sauce 1 teaspoon honey

A pinch of salt

1 teaspoon gochugaru (Korean red chili pepper flakes)

Directions

Start by preheating your Air Fryer to 380 degrees F. Spritz the Air Fryer basket with cooking oil.

Mix the salmon, egg, garlic, green onions, and rolled oats in a bowl; knead with your hands until everything is well incorporated.

Shape the mixture into equally sized patties. Transfer your patties to the Air Fryer basket.

Cook the fish patties for 10 minutes, turning them over halfway through.

Meanwhile, make the sauce by whisking all Ingredients. Serve the warm fish patties with the sauce on the side.

Monkfish Fillets with Romano Cheese

(Ready in about 15 minutes | Servings 2)

Per serving:

415 Calories; 22.5g Fat; 3.7g Carbs; 47.4g Protein; 2.3g Sugars

Ingredients

2 monkfish fillets

1 teaspoon garlic paste

2 tablespoons butter, melted

1/2 teaspoon Aleppo chili powder 1/2 teaspoon dried rosemary

1/4 teaspoon cracked black pepper

1/2 teaspoon sea salt

4 tablespoons Romano cheese, grated

Directions

Start by preheating the Air Fryer to 320 degrees F. Spritz the Air Fryer basket with cooking oil.

Spread the garlic paste all over the fish fillets.

Brush the monkfish fillets with the melted butter on both sides. Sprinkle with the chili powder, rosemary, black pepper, and salt. Cook for 7 minutes in the preheated Air Fryer.

Top with the Romano cheese and continue to cook for 2 minutes more or until heated through. Bon appétit!

Monkfish with Sautéed Vegetables and Olives

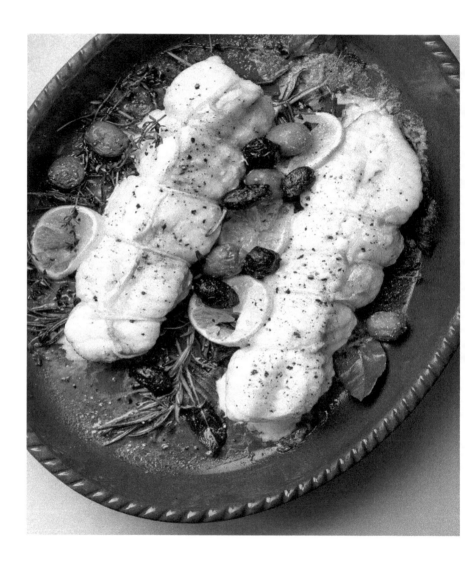

(Ready in about 20 minutes | Servings 2)

Per serving:

310 Calories; 13.3g Fat; 12.7g Carbs; 35.2g Protein; 5.4g Sugars

Ingredients

2 teaspoons olive oil 2 carrots, sliced

2 bell peppers, sliced

1 teaspoon dried thyme

1/2 teaspoon dried marjoram 1/2 teaspoon dried rosemary 2 monkfish fillets

1 tablespoon soy sauce 2 tablespoons lime juice

Coarse salt and ground black pepper, to taste 1 teaspoon cayenne pepper

1/2 cup Kalamata olives, pitted and sliced

Directions

In a nonstick skillet, heat the olive oil for 1 minute. Once hot, sauté the carrots and peppers until tender, about 4 minutes. Sprinkle with thyme, marjoram, and rosemary and set aside.

Toss the fish fillets with the soy sauce, lime juice, salt, black pepper, and cayenne pepper. Place the fish fillets in a lightly greased cooking basket and bake at 390 degrees F for 8 minutes.

Turn them over, add the olives, and cook an additional 4 minutes. Serve with the sautéed vegetables on the side. Bon appétit!

Old Bay Calamari

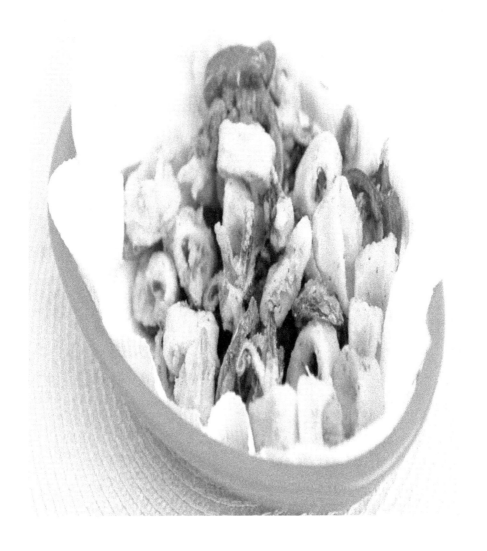

(Ready in about 20 minutes + marinating time | Servings 3)

Per serving:

448 Calories; 5.3g Fat; 58.9g Carbs; 31.9g Protein; 0.2g Sugars

Ingredients

1 cup beer

1 pound squid, cleaned and cut into rings 1 cup all-purpose flour

2 eggs

1/2 cup cornstarch Sea salt, to taste

1/2 teaspoon ground black pepper 1 tablespoon Old Bay seasoning

Directions

Add the beer and squid in a glass bowl, cover and let it sit in your refrigerator for 1 hour.

Preheat your Air Fryer to 390 degrees F. Rinse the squid and pat it dry.

Place the flour in a shallow bowl. In another bowl, whisk the eggs. Add the cornstarch and seasonings to a third shallow bowl.

Dredge the calamari in the flour. Then, dip them into the egg mixture; finally, coat them with the cornstarch on all sided.

Arrange them in the cooking basket. Spritz with cooking oil and cook for 9 to 12 minutes, depending on the desired level of doneness. Work in batches.

Serve warm with your favorite dipping sauce. Enjoy!

Quick-Fix Seafood Breakfast

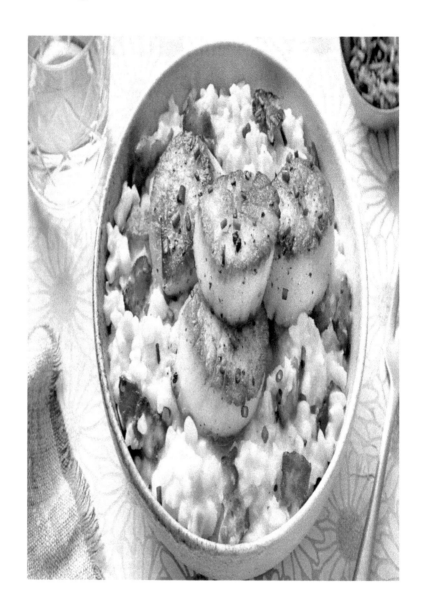

(Ready in about 30 minutes | Servings 2)

Per serving:

414 Calories; 23.4g Fat; 11.6g Carbs; 38.8g Protein; 7.2g Sugars

Ingredients

1 tablespoon olive oil 2 garlic cloves, minced

1 small yellow onion, chopped

1/4 pound tilapia pieces 1/4 pound rockfish pieces 1/2 teaspoon dried basil

Salt and white pepper, to taste 4 eggs, lightly beaten

1 tablespoon dry sherry

4 tablespoons cheese, shredded

Directions

Start by preheating your Air Fryer to 350 degrees F; add the olive oil to a baking pan. Once hot, cook the garlic and onion for 2 minutes or until fragrant.

Add the fish, basil, salt, and pepper. In a mixing dish, thoroughly combine the eggs with sherry and cheese. Pour the mixture into the baking pan.

Cook at 360 degrees F approximately 20 minutes. Bon appétit!

Salmon Filets with Fennel Slaw

(Ready in about 15 minutes | Servings 3)

Per serving:

337 Calories; 13.6g Fat; 19.3g Carbs; 36.3g Protein; 8.2g Sugars

Ingredients

1 pound salmon filets

1 teaspoon Cajun spice mix

Sea salt and ground black pepper, to taste Fennel Slaw:

1 pound fennel bulb, thinly sliced 1 Lebanese cucumber, thinly sliced 1/2 red onion, thinly sliced

1/2 ounce tarragon 2 tablespoons tahini

2 tablespoons lemon juice 1 tablespoon soy sauce

Directions

Rinse the salmon filets and pat them dry with a paper towel. Then, toss the salmon filets with the Cajun spice mix, salt and black pepper.

Cook the salmon filets in the preheated Air Fryer at 380 degrees F for 6 minutes; flip the salmon filets and cook for a further 6 minutes.

Meanwhile, make the fennel slaw by stirring fennel, cucumber, red onion and tarragon in a salad bowl. Mix the remaining Ingredients to make the dressing.

Dress the salad and transfer to your refrigerator until ready to serve. Serve the warm fish with chilled fennel slaw. Bon appétit!

Salmon with Baby Bok Choy

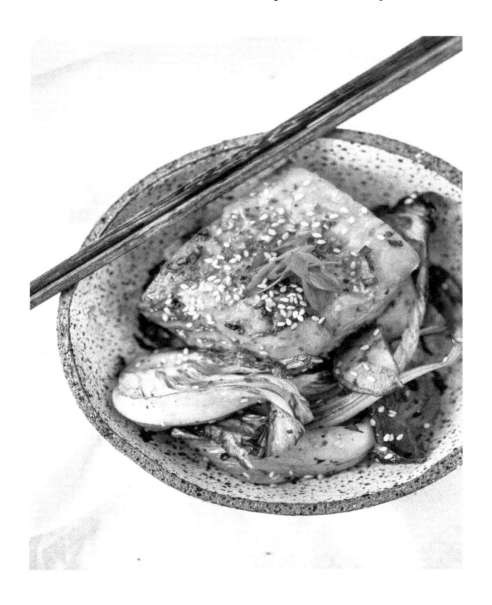

(Ready in about 20 minutes | Servings 3)

Per serving:

308 Calories; 13.6g Fat; 12.2g Carbs; 34.3g Protein; 9.3g Sugars

Ingredients

1 pound salmon filets

1 teaspoon garlic chili paste 1 teaspoon sesame oil

1 tablespoon honey

1 tablespoon soy sauce

1 pound baby Bok choy, bottoms removed Kosher salt and black pepper, to taste

Directions

Start by preheating your Air Fryer to 380 degrees F.

Toss the salmon fillets with garlic chili paste, sesame oil, honey, soy sauce, salt and black pepper.

Cook the salmon in the preheated Air Fryer for 6 minutes; turn the filets over and cook an additional 6 minutes.

Then, cook the baby Bok choy at 350 degrees F for 3 minutes; shake the basket and cook an additional 3 minutes. Salt and pepper to taste.

Serve the salmon fillets with the roasted baby Bok choy. Enjoy!

Saucy Garam Masala Fish

(Ready in about 25 minutes | Servings 2)

Per serving:

301 Calories; 12.1g Fat; 2.3g Carbs; 43g Protein; 1.6g Sugars

Ingredients

2 teaspoons olive oil 1/4 cup coconut milk

1/2 teaspoon cayenne pepper

1 teaspoon Garam masala

1/4 teaspoon Kala namak (Indian black salt) 1/2 teaspoon fresh ginger, grated

1 garlic clove, minced 2 catfish fillets

1/4 cup coriander, roughly chopped

Directions

Preheat your Air Fryer to 390 degrees F. Then, spritz the baking dish with a nonstick cooking spray.

In a mixing bowl, whisk the olive oil, milk, cayenne pepper, Garam masala, Kala namak, ginger, and garlic.

Coat the catfish fillets with the Garam masala mixture. Cook the catfish fillets in the preheated Air Fryer approximately 18 minutes, turning over halfway through the cooking time.

Garnish with fresh coriander and serve over hot noodles if desired.

Scallops with Pineapple Salsa and Pickled Onions

(Ready in about 15 minutes | Servings 3)

Per serving:

177 Calories; 2.6g Fat; 22.3g Carbs; 15.6g Protein; 15g Sugars

Ingredients

12 scallops

1 teaspoon sesame oil

1/4 teaspoon dried rosemary 1/2 teaspoon dried tarragon 1/2 teaspoon dried basil

1/4 teaspoon red pepper flakes, crushed Coarse sea salt and black pepper, to taste 1/2 cup pickled onions, drained Pineapple Salsa:

1 cup pineapple, diced

2 tablespoons fresh cilantro, roughly chopped 1 jalapeño, deveined and minced

1 small-sized red onion, minced

1 teaspoon ginger root, peeled and grated 1/2 teaspoon coconut sugar

Sea salt and ground black pepper, to taste

Directions

Toss the scallops sesame oil, rosemary, tarragon, basil, red pepper, salt and black pepper.

Cook in the preheated Air Fryer at 400 degrees F for 6 to 7 minutes, shaking the basket once or twice to ensure even cooking.

Meanwhile, process all the salsa Ingredients in your blender; cover and place the salsa in your refrigerator until ready to serve.

Serve the warm scallops with pickled onions and pineapple salsa on the side. Bon appétit!

Seed-Crusted Codfish Fillets

(Ready in about 15 minutes | Servings 2)

Per serving:

263 Calories; 8.3g Fat; 8.2g Carbs; 37.7g Protein; 1.2g Sugars

Ingredients

2 codfish fillets

1 teaspoon sesame oil

Sea salt and black pepper, to taste 1 teaspoon sesame seeds

1 tablespoon chia seeds

Directions

Start by preheating your Air Fryer to 380 degrees F.

Add the sesame oil, salt, black pepper, sesame seeds and chia seeds to a rimmed plate. Coat the top of the codfish with the seed mixture, pressing it down to adhere.

Lower the codfish fillets, seed side down, into the cooking basket and cook for 6 minutes. Turn the fish fillets over and cook for a further 6 minutes.

Serve warm and enjoy!

Shrimp Scampi Linguine

(Ready in about 25 minutes | Servings 4)

Per serving:

560 Calories; 15.1g Fat; 47.3g Carbs; 59.3g Protein; 1.6g Sugars

1 ½ pounds shrimp, shelled and deveined 1/2 tablespoon fresh basil leaves, chopped 2 tablespoons olive oil

2 cloves garlic, minced

1/2 teaspoon fresh ginger, grated 1/4 teaspoon cracked black pepper 1/2 teaspoon sea salt

1/4 cup chicken stock 2 ripe tomatoes, pureed 8 ounces linguine pasta

1/2 cup parmesan cheese, preferably freshly grated

Directions

Start by preheating the Air Fryer to 395 degrees F. Place the shrimp, basil, olive oil, garlic, ginger, black pepper, salt, chicken stock, and tomatoes in the casserole dish.

Transfer the casserole dish to the cooking basket and bake for 10 minutes.

Bring a large pot of lightly salted water to a boil. Cook the linguine for 10 minutes or until al dente; drain.

Divide between four serving plates. Add the shrimp sauce and top with parmesan cheese. Bon appétit!

Smoked Halibut and Eggs in Brioche

(Ready in about 25 minutes | Servings 4)

Per serving:

372 Calories; 13.1g Fat; 22g Carbs; 38.6g Protein; 3.3g Sugars

Ingredients

4 brioche rolls

1 pound smoked halibut, chopped 4 eggs

1 teaspoon dried thyme 1 teaspoon dried basil

Salt and black pepper, to taste

Directions

Cut off the top of each brioche; then, scoop out the insides to make the shells.

Lay the prepared brioche shells in the lightly greased cooking basket.

Spritz with cooking oil; add the halibut. Crack an egg into each brioche shell; sprinkle with thyme, basil, salt, and black pepper.

Bake in the preheated Air Fryer at 325 degrees F for 20 minutes. Bon appétit!

Snapper Casserole with Gruyere Cheese

(Ready in about 25 minutes | Servings 4)

Per serving:

406 Calories; 19.9g Fat; 9.3g Carbs; 46.4g Protein; 4.5g Sugars

Ingredients

2 tablespoons olive oil 1 shallot, thinly sliced 2 garlic cloves, minced

1 ½ pounds snapper fillets

Sea salt and ground black pepper, to taste 1 teaspoon cayenne pepper

1/2 teaspoon dried basil 1/2 cup tomato puree 1/2 cup white wine

1 cup Gruyere cheese, shredded

Directions

Heat 1 tablespoon of olive oil in a saucepan over medium-high heat. Now, cook the shallot and garlic until tender and aromatic.

Preheat your Air Fryer to 370 degrees F.

Grease a casserole dish with 1 tablespoon of olive oil. Place the snapper fillet in the casserole dish. Season with salt, black pepper, and cayenne pepper.

Add the sautéed shallot mixture.

Add the basil, tomato puree and wine to the casserole dish. Cook for 10 minutes in the preheated Air Fryer.

Top with the shredded cheese and cook an additional 7 minutes. Serve immediately.

Spicy Curried King Prawns

(Ready in about 10 minutes | Servings 2)

Per serving:

220 Calories; 9.7g Fat; 15.1g Carbs; 17.6g Protein; 2.2g Sugars

Ingredients

12 king prawns, rinsed 1 tablespoon coconut oil

1/2 teaspoon piri piri powder

Salt and ground black pepper, to taste 1 teaspoon garlic paste

1 teaspoon onion powder

1/2 teaspoon cumin powder 1 teaspoon curry powder

Directions

In a mixing bowl, toss all ingredient until the prawns are well coated on all sides.

Cook in the preheated Air Fryer at 360 degrees F for 4 minutes. Shake the basket and cook for 4 minutes more.

Serve over hot rice if desired. Bon appétit!

Sunday Fish with Sticky Sauce

(Ready in about 20 minutes | Servings 2)

Per serving:

573 Calories; 38.3g Fat; 31.5g Carbs; 26.2g Protein; 5.7g Sugars

Ingredients

2 pollack fillets

Salt and black pepper, to taste 1 tablespoon olive oil

1 cup chicken broth

2 tablespoons light soy sauce 1 tablespoon brown sugar

2 tablespoons butter, melted

1 teaspoon fresh ginger, minced 1 teaspoon fresh garlic, minced 2 corn tortillas

Directions

Pat dry the pollack fillets and season them with salt and black pepper; drizzle the sesame oil all over the fish fillets.

Preheat the Air Fryer to 380 degrees F and cook your fish for 11 minutes. Slice into bite-sized pieces.

Meanwhile, prepare the sauce. Add the broth to a large saucepan and bring to a boil. Add the soy sauce, sugar, butter, ginger, and garlic. Reduce the heat to simmer and cook until it is reduced slightly.

Add the fish pieces to the warm sauce. Serve on corn tortillas and enjoy!

Swordfish with Roasted Peppers and Garlic Sauce

(Ready in about 30 minutes | Servings 3)

Per serving:

274 Calories; 14.1g Fat; 5.1g Carbs; 30.5g Protein; 3.2g Sugars

Ingredients

3 bell peppers

3 swordfish steaks

1 tablespoon butter, melted 2 garlic cloves, minced

Sea salt and freshly ground black pepper, to taste 1/2 teaspoon cayenne pepper

1/2 teaspoon ginger powder

Directions

Start by preheating your Air Fryer to 400 degrees F. Brush the Air Fryer basket lightly with cooking oil.

Then, roast the bell peppers for 5 minutes. Give the peppers a half turn; place them back in the cooking basket and roast for another 5 minutes.

Turn them one more time and roast until the skin is charred and soft or 5 more minutes. Peel the peppers and set aside.

Then, add the swordfish steaks to the lightly greased cooking basket and cook at 400 degrees F for 10 minutes.

Meanwhile, melt the butter in a small saucepan. Cook the garlic until fragrant and add the salt, pepper, cayenne pepper, and ginger powder. Cook until everything is thoroughly heated.

Plate the peeled peppers and the roasted swordfish; spoon the sauce over them and serve warm.

Tortilla-Crusted Haddock Fillets

(Ready in about 20 minutes | Servings 2)

Per serving:

384 Calories; 21.3g Fat; 7.6g Carbs; 38.4g Protein; 1g Sugars

Ingredients

2 haddock fillets

1/2 cup tortilla chips, crushed

2 tablespoons parmesan cheese, freshly grated 1 teaspoon dried parsley flakes

1 egg, beaten

1/2 teaspoon coarse sea salt

1/4 teaspoon ground black pepper 1/4 teaspoon cayenne pepper

2 tablespoons olive oil

Directions

Start by preheating your Air Fryer to 360 degrees F. Pat dry the haddock fillets and set aside.

In a shallow bowl, thoroughly combine the crushed tortilla chips with the parmesan and parsley flakes. Mix until everything is well incorporated.

In a separate shallow bowl, whisk the egg with salt, black pepper, and cayenne pepper.

Dip the haddock fillets into the egg. Then, dip the fillets into the tortilla/parmesan mixture until well coated on all sides.

Drizzle the olive oil all over the fish fillets. Lower the coated fillets into the lightly greased Air Fryer basket. Cook for 11 to 13 minutes. Bon appétit!

Tuna Steak with Roasted Cherry Tomatoes

(Ready in about 15 minutes | Servings 2)

Per serving:

231 Calories; 3.3g Fat; 6.2g Carbs; 45.2g Protein; 3.7g Sugars

Ingredients

1 pound tuna steak

1 cup cherry tomatoes

1 teaspoon extra-virgin olive oil

2 sprigs rosemary, leaves picked and crushed Sea salt and red pepper flakes, to taste

1 teaspoon garlic, finely chopped

1 tablespoon lime juice

Directions

Toss the tuna steaks and cherry tomatoes with olive oil, rosemary leaves, salt, black pepper and garlic.

Place the tuna steaks in a lightly oiled cooking basket; cook tuna steaks at 440 degrees F for about 6 minutes.

Turn the tuna steaks over, add in the cherry tomatoes and continue to cook for 4 minutes more. Drizzle the fish with lime juice and serve warm garnished with roasted cherry tomatoes!

Tuna Steaks with Pearl Onions

(Ready in about 20 minutes | Servings 4)

Per serving:

332 Calories; 5.9g Fat; 10.5g Carbs; 56.1g Protein; 6.1g Sugars

Ingredients

4 tuna steaks

1 pound pearl onions 4 teaspoons olive oil

1 teaspoon dried rosemary 1 teaspoon dried marjoram

1 tablespoon cayenne pepper

1/2 teaspoon sea salt

1/2 teaspoon black pepper, preferably freshly cracked 1 lemon, sliced

Directions

Place the tuna steaks in the lightly greased cooking basket. Top with the pearl onions; add the olive oil, rosemary, marjoram, cayenne pepper, salt, and black pepper.

Bake in the preheated Air Fryer at 400 degrees F for 9 to 10 minutes. Work in two batches.

Serve warm with lemon slices and enjoy!

Vermouth and Garlic Shrimp Skewers

(Ready in about 15 minutes + marinating time | Servings 4)

Per serving:

371 Calories; 12.2g Fat; 30.4g Carbs; 29.5g Protein; 3.2g Sugars

Ingredients

1 ½ pounds shrimp 1/4 cup vermouth

2 cloves garlic, crushed

1 teaspoon dry mango powder Kosher salt, to taste

1/4 teaspoon black pepper, freshly ground

2 tablespoons olive oil 4 tablespoons flour

8 skewers, soaked in water for 30 minutes

1 lemon, cut into wedges

Directions

Add the shrimp, vermouth, garlic, mango powder, salt, black pepper, and olive oil in a ceramic bowl; let it sit for 1 hour in your refrigerator.

Discard the marinade and toss the shrimp with flour. Thread on to skewers and transfer to the lightly greased cooking basket.

Cook at 400 degrees F for 5 minutes, tossing halfway through. Serve with lemon wedges. Bon appétit!

Alphabetical Index

A

Authentic Mediterranean Calamari Salad...1

Alphabetical Index...104

B

Buttermilk Tuna fillets 3

C

Cajun Cod Fillets with Avocado Sauce..6

Cajun Fish Cakes with Cheese 9

Coconut Shrimp with Orange Sauce 12

Cod and Shallot Frittata..15

Crab Cake Burgers 17

Crispy Mustardy Fish Fingers 20

Crispy Tilapia Fillets...23

D

Delicious Snapper en Papillote..26

Dilled and Glazed Salmon Steaks 29

E

Easy Lobster Tails 32

Easy Prawns alla Parmigiana..35

English-Style Flounder Fillets...38

G

Greek-Style Roast Fish...41

Grilled Hake with Garlic Sauce...44

Grilled Salmon Steaks 47

Grilled Tilapia with Portobello Mushrooms...50

H

Halibut Cakes with Horseradish Mayo...53

I

Indian Famous Fish Curry 56

K

Korean-Style Salmon Patties 59

M

Monkfish Fillets with Romano Cheese 62

Monkfish with Sautéed Vegetables and Olives 64

O

Old Bay Calamari 67

Q

Quick-Fix Seafood Breakfast 70

S

Salmon Filets with Fennel Slaw 73

Salmon with Baby Bok Choy 75

Saucy Garam Masala Fish 78

Scallops with Pineapple Salsa and Pickled Onions 80

Seed-Crusted Codfish Fillets 82

Shrimp Scampi Linguine 84

Smoked Halibut and Eggs in Brioche..86

Snapper Casserole with Gruyere Cheese...88

Spicy Curried King Prawns 90

Sunday Fish with Sticky Sauce 92

Swordfish with Roasted Peppers and Garlic Sauce......................................94

T

Tortilla-Crusted Haddock Fillets 96

Tuna Steak with Roasted Cherry Tomatoes 98

Tuna Steaks with Pearl Onions...100

V

Vermouth and Garlic Shrimp Skewers 102

CPSIA information can be obtained
at www.ICGtesting.com
Printed in the USA
LVHW020946050521
686547LV00008B/683